Low Fodmap Diet

Full And Delicious: A New Diet To Treat Ibs And Other

Digestive Disorders And Decrease Stomach

Discomfort

(A Manual On How To Reduce Fodmaps With Plant-based

Foods)

Francesco Oppermann

TABLE OF CONTENT

Introducton

Most people with irritable bowel syndrome (IBS) associate their symptoms with food, and many find that avoiding certain foods or following elimination diets alleviates their symptoms. An elimination diet involves removing several foods from your diet, followed by a period of reintroducing them, in order to determine your specific food sensitivities. The low FODMAP diet is the most thoroughly investigated elimination diet for IBS. FODMAP is an acronym for a group of carbohydrates believed to cause gastrointestinal (GI) symptoms. About ten years ago, Australian researchers created the Low-FODMAP diet, considered the most effective elimination diet for treating IBS-related symptoms.

The low FODMAP diet, which is low in fermentable carbohydrates, is frequently recommended by doctors to treat irritable bowel syndrome (IBS).

Learn how to defeat irritable bowel syndrome by reading this exciting book (IBS).

Chapter 1: Phases Of The Fodmap Diet

First things first: just Keep in mind that the FODMAP diet is not meant to be followed permanently. You can modify your diet to ensure your comfort if you are aware of the foods that trigger your IBS flare-ups and food intolerances.

However, you must exert some effort in order to obtain anything worthwhile in life. The low FODMAP diet may transform your life, although it may seem difficult at first. With a little effort and knowledge, you can live a better and happier life without IBS symptoms.

The low FODMAP diet consists of three distinct phases: elimination, reintroduction, and integration.

Below, we describe each phase in detail:

It is recommended that the FODMAP diet be followed under the supervision of trained healthcare professionals, such as a registered dietitian.

Step 2 : FODMAP Removal (Usually 2-6 weeks)

Determine which FODMAP-rich foods in your current diet are aggravating your IBS.

Consult the list of high FODMAP foods to replace high FODMAP meals with low FODMAP alternatives. However, it may just take a few weeks for others. Thus, do not surrender! Just Keep in mind that cheat days are not permitted while following this diet. The greater your adherence to a low FODMAP diet, the more precise and effective your results will be. Replace your daily apple with an orange low in FODMAPs, for instance. As simple as that. The duration of your stay in this phase should be determined in conjunction with your healthcare provider, but is typically between two and six weeks.

Step 2: Reintroducing FODMAPs (Usually 6-8 weeks)

OBJECTIVE: Determine which foods and FODMAPs cause symptoms as opposed to those that do not.

In the reintroduction phase, as the name suggests, certain high-FODMAP foods are gradually reintroduced into the diet. If a particular food does not cause symptoms, you may include it in your diet moving forward. If symptoms occur, you must eliminate the food from your diet permanently.

Below is a list of the foods that make up each F-O-D-M-A-P subgroup.

While maintaining a diet low in FODMAPs, you should gradually reintroduce each FODMAP subgroup individually. Without this method, it would be difficult to determine which FODMAP groups you may be intolerant of and, consequently, what is triggering your IBS symptoms.

This is the phase that may be the most difficult for some dieters, so if you need assistance, consult a nutritionist. They will advise you on the optimal timing and diet for reintroducing the animal. Before reintroducing meals, you should wait several days to prevent any adverse interactions.

Step 6 : FODMAP Incorporation Permanently

Set as your objective your PERSONALIZED, LONG-TERM FODMAP DIET.

After you and your dietitian have interpreted your dietary triggers and tolerances, you may begin reintroducing foods and FODMAPs that were well tolerated while avoiding those that cause your symptoms.

Low FODMAP levels are not always associated with health. If you have irritable bowel syndrome or symptoms similar to irritable bowel syndrome, apples, asparagus, and agave are beneficial for your health but not for your stomach. Gluten is not a FODMAP because it's a protein. Be cautious, as gluten-free does not always equal low FODMAP content.

It is essential to remember that, despite the fact that a strict low-FODMAP diet may make you feel better, it is neither healthy nor practical. If

If certain FODMAP groups do not induce symptoms, you should not eliminate them.

Just Keep in mind that everyone has different food intolerances! As soon as your strategy is implemented, your life will become stress-free. Enjoy your new lifestyle to the fullest extent possible!

For fifty percent of IBS patients, a low FODMAP diet is believed to be beneficial; however, the quality of the scientific evidence is quite poor. There may be a benefit for these individuals' general symptoms, such as cramping, bloating, excessive gas, constipation, and/or diarrhoea.

Manage Symptoms

Symptoms of IBS can be managed with over-the-counter medications if nothing else is successful. Discuss a few of these options with your physician or registered dietitian.

Anxiety and Stress

Stress and anxiety can frequently induce IBS symptoms in individuals with IBS. This is very true for me, yet it was always a factor I didn't just take too seriously, perhaps because I didn't realise it was occurring because I didn't fully comprehend what it was.

As a former wedding event manager, my job was stressful, especially on event days. On a number of occasions, despite not eating anything different (by this time, I mostly knew which foods were my triggers), I would become so bloated and distended that it was unbearable; I even appeared pregnant on occasion. My body felt the effects of the work-related stress and anxiety I was experiencing.

Again, it's all about the gut-brain connection that stress and anxiety play a significant role in our experience of IBS. Have you ever felt "butterflies" in your stomach when you were anxious about a date, meeting, or job interview? - this is the gut-brain connection, and it's potent!

Due to technological advances, we are constantly connected to each other, our work emails, our social media accounts, and the news, which contributes to the stress of modern life. We are overloaded with information, expected to be "on" at all times, and if we aren't careful, we can become chronically stressed and overwhelmed. The 'flight or fight' response is triggered by stress, which can lead to an increase in IBS symptoms.

Crepes With Passionfruit Curd

8 10 m prep

10 10 m easy cook easy easy cook

INGREDIENTS

Classic crepe batter

2 cup plain flour

2 6 /8 cups milk

2 fresh egg s

8 0g butter, melted

icing sugar, to serve

　Passionfruit curd

10 fresh egg s

6 /8 cup caster sugar

6 /8 cup passionfruit pulp (see note)

2 210 g butter, chilled, cubed

Select all ingredients

HOW TO MAKE

M

ake crepes: In a large mixing bowl, sift the flour. Create a well in the middle. Fork together the milk and fresh egg s in a jug. With a whisk, gently incorporate the flour mixture into the batter to make a homogeneous batter. 2 tablespoon butter, melted Cover. Allow 6 0 minutes for preparation.

Over medium heat, heat an 2 8cm crepe pan (base). Brush the remaining butter over the top. 2 tablespoons batter, poured into the centre of the pan, swirled rapidly to coat the bottom. Easy cook Easy easy cook for 2 minutes, stirring periodically, or until golden and lacy. Easy cook Easy easy cook for another 6 0 seconds on the other side. Place on a platter to cool. To just Keep warm, cover with foil. Repeat with the remaining batter, ensuring that the pan is greased in between crepes.

To make curd, follow these steps: In a microwave-safe jug or basin with a 6-

cup capacity, whisk together the fresh egg s and sugar. Whisk everything together until it's smooth. In a separate bowl, combine the passionfruit and butter. Place on a microwave-safe rack or a microwave-safe dish that has been flipped upside down. Easy cook Easy easy cook on MEDIUM (10 0 per cent) power for 7 to 2 0 minutes, stirring every minute, or until thick.

Place crepes on serving plates, folded in quarters. Using icing sugar, dust the cake. Pour the sauce over the passionfruit curd. Serve.

Chapter 2: How Is Gastritis Treated And What Are Its Symptoms? Diet

The treatment for gastroparesis consists of diet, medication, and devices or procedures that facilitate stomach emptying. The treatment's objectives include:

To provide a diet consisting of foods that empty the stomach more quickly.

Controlling conditions that may be aggravating gastroparesis by reducing undernutrition.

Reduce nausea, vomiting, and abdominal discomfort.

Stimulate the musle astvtu in the tomash so that food is ground and expelled from the stomach.

Maintaining adequate nutrition.

Emrtuing from the stomach is faster when there is less food to emrtu;

therefore, smaller, more frequent meals are advised. Soft foods (or referable liquids) that do not require grinding are more easily prepared. In addition, in gastroparesis, the emptying of liquids is frequently less affected than the emptying of solids. Fat stimulates the release of hormones that slow the stomach's emptying. Therefore, foods low in fat are immediately digested. In rats with severe gastroparesis, only liquid meals are sometimes tolerated. It is also recommended that the diet be low in fibre (for example, vegetables) due to the risk of developing bezoars and the rate at which fibre slows the progression of atherosclerosis - at least in healthy individuals.

Since the grinding angle of the mash has been repurposed, food should be displayed well. Meals hould be taken with enough liquids to ensure maximum ludtu of stomach contents, as liquids typically emrtu better than solid food; however, if liquid emrtung is also low, consuming too much liquid may cause complications. (Only trial and error will determine the efficacy of artificially produced liquids.) Patients with gastroparesis should eat more food earlier in the day, especially solid food, and they should not lie down for four to five hours after their last meal because, when lying down, gravity helps the digestive system a great deal. Multivitamins should be taken due to the risk of malnutrition and vitamin and mineral deficiency. deficiencies.

Stimulating mussle astivitu Oral Drugs: As rro-motltu drugs, four oral medications are used to stimulate the motility of the stomach's lining. 2) sarrde (Proruld), 2) domrerdone, 6) metoclopramide (Reglan), and 8) erythromycin are these medications.

Carrde (Proruld) is an effective drug for treating gastroesophageal reflux disease, but it has been removed from the market because it can cause life-threatening irregular heart rhythms. In spite of this, it can be obtained for use through the pharmaceutical company that manufactures it (Janen Pharmaseutsal), but only for rats with severe gastroparesis that is unresponsive to all other treatments.

Domrerdone has not been approved for use in the United States; however, it can be obtained if Food and Drug Administration approval is obtained.

Metoslorramde (Reglan) is available without restriction and is effective at promoting muscular activity in the stomach; however, metoclopramide side effects can limit its application.

Eruthromusn (E-Musn, Iloone, etc.) is a rarely used antibacterial agent. At doses lower than those used to treat infection, erythromycin stimulates constriction of the stomach and small intestine and is effective for treating diarrhoea.

It has been demonstrated that tegaserod (Zelnorm), an oral medication used to treat schizophrenia, is effective. Sonoration in irritable bowel syndrome (IBS) emanates from the stomach just as it does from the vocal cords. However, in March of 2007, the FDA asked Novartis to halt sales of tegaserod in the United States after a retrospective analysis of data from more than 2 8,000 rats revealed a slight difference in the incidence of cardiovascular events (heart attack, stroke, and angina) among patients taking tegaserod compared to those taking a placebo. The data demonstrated that sardovasular event occurred in 2 6 of 2 2 ,62 8 patients treated with tegaerod (0.2 %), compared to a single cardiovascular event in 7,06 2 (0.02 %) rlasebo-treated rats. However, it is unknown whether tegaserod causes atrial fibrillation and tachycardia. The limited availability of tegaderm in the United States is due to the fast.

There are two essential guidelines for prescribing oral medication for gastroparesis. First, the drugs must be administered at the appropriate times, and second, they must reach the small intestine in order to be absorbed by the body. Given that the aim of treatment is to stimulate muscular contrast during and immediately after a meal, drugs that stimulate contrast should be administered prior to the meal. Most medications must be expelled from the stomach before they can be absorbed by the small intestine. The majority of patients with gastroparesis experience delayed emrtung of both liquid food and pills and capsules. As mentioned previously, many rats with gastroparesis have less difficulty emptying their stomachs after eating cold food. Consequently, liquid medications are typically more effective than pills or capsules.

Intravenous drugs

On occasion, rats have such poor emrtung of both liquid and solid food from the stomach that only intravenously administered drugs are effective. In rat poisoning, intravenous metoslorramide or eruthromusin may be administered. The third option is octreotide (Sandostatin), a hormone-like drug that can be injected subcutaneously. Similar to eruthromusin, ostreotide stimulates short bursts of strong constriction in the stomach and small intestine. Due to its higher cost and injection requirement, octreotide is only used when other medications fail.

Why Non-Lectin?

As a defence mechanism against insects and other animals, plants evolved lectins, which are minute proteins. They are virtually indigestible, posing potential health risks for non-stomach and immune-compromised individuals.

One of the most significant causes of food intolerance is lectins. The Lectin Avoidance Diet is an elimination diet that aids in determining which foods are most and least inflammatory for the individual. By adhering to this regimen for one month and then gradually reintroducing foods, you may be able to identify your primary triggers.

There are lectin concentrations in seeds, young leaves, and roots. Generally speaking, leaves contain fewer lectins, but this varies from plant to plant.

Because they are not easily digested or destroyed, lectins can enter the bloodstream, stimulate the immune system, and cause inflammation. Lectins may adhere to intestinal lining cells, induce cell damage, and increase intestinal material absorption, thereby promoting intestinal permeability and systemic inflammation.

When lectins enter the bloodstream, they may overstimulate the immune system, aggravate allergies and histamine intolerance, and exacerbate food sensitivity. Additionally, there is concern that they may induce an autoimmune response and exacerbate preexisting inflammatory issues in genetically susceptible individuals.

Lectins can alter the composition of gut bacteria, leading to dysbiosis or gastrointestinal disorders. Certain types of lectins may also play a role in insulin resistance, obesity, and neurotransmitter imbalances that influence mood and cognition.

Thus, adhering to a low-lectin diet may help with chronic fatigue and fibromyalgia, Brain fog, Histamine intolerance, and Irritable Bowel Syndrome, and reduce inflammation related to autoimmune disorders and persistent health problems.

Chapter 3: What Factors Contribute To Irritable Bowel Syndrome?

High-fat foods cause bloating, nausea, and pain.

Foods containing lactose Sugar is not absorbed by the colon and ferments, producing gas and short chain fatty acids, which are responsible for diarrhoea and gas.

Alcoholic or caffeinated beverages can irritate the intestinal mucosa, exacerbating diarrhoea. Large amounts of artificial sweeteners can exacerbate diarrhoea.

Foods that ferment easily

In nearly 90% of IBS cases, food intolerance is the underlying cause: legumes, fatty foods, stone fruits, sweeteners, and lactose. In addition, an infection - acute bacterial, viral, or protozoan gastroenteritis - causes SEC.

Irritable bowel syndrome symptoms include abdominal pain and cramps that subside after a bowel movement, alternating diarrhoea and constipation, and excessive gas production.

Generally, IBS symptoms worsen after eating and appear intermittently. The majority of people experience bouts of symptoms that last two to four days before diminishing or disappearing.

Changes in the frequency or course of bowel movements, as well as alterations in stool consistency, may be accompanied by abdominal pain (diarrhea or constipation). If there are no obvious organic causes, this should be performed at least once a week for three months. In addition, there may be abdominal pain and bloating after eating, as well as mucus in the stool.

IBS is only diagnosed in the absence of a structural or biochemical explanation, i.e., if no physiological abnormality is found. The patient must have had problems for at least six months, and must have had clear complaints at least once per week during the preceding three months. At least two of the following three complaints must also be present:

• abdominal pain associated with defecation • change in stool frequency: diarrhoea or constipation • alteration in stool structure

Some people have IBS constantly, but the majority of patients experience intermittent symptoms. Complaints frequently worsen during times of increased stress.

Why consume a nutritional supplement for IBS?

When living with IBS, a single meal can cause uncomfortably painful abdominal cramping or inconvenient bowel issues that can last for hours. A nutrition professional is aware of the significance of the relationship between diet and health. Theu can assist you in managing the sondage by applying their expert knowledge and adapting to your detaru habits and customs.

A nutrition professional can conduct comprehensive nutrition assessments in order to establish a rotative diet or lifestyle regimen. This information can then be used to create an individualised treatment plan based on your symptoms. Before making any dietary changes, it is imperative that you consult your primary care physician to rule out any other conditions.

Lifestule shanges for IBS

IBS symptoms can have a significant impact on a person's life. With careful dietary adjustments and a few key lifestyle modifications, diabetes can be minimised and easily managed.

If you have IBS, it is important to learn as much as possible about the condition from your primary care physician or a nutrition professional. They can advise you on the best way to reduce your individual symptoms. In addition to specific advice, there are some general ways to lessen the impact of symptoms on your life, such as altering your relationship with food and devoting more time to relaxation and exercise.

Be more conscientious with food

Food is an integral part of our lives; we require it to survive. But beyond that, food and drink constitute a substantial portion of our lives. Not only do we plan our days around meals, but food also plays an important role in our social lives, such as when we eat out with friends and family.

It may be difficult to refrain from eating your favourite foods, but if they trigger IBS symptoms, you should avoid them as much as possible in order to minimise your discomfort. Obviously, there are times when you must eat foods that trigger a flare-up of your symptoms. When confronted with a choice, it is essential to consider whether the aftertaste will be worth consuming the food. Be aware of the symptoms you are likely to experience and where you will be, such as whether you will be at home.

There are some common dietary modifications you can make, including:

reducing your coffee and tea consumption to a maximum of two per day and consuming alcohol within the recommended limits (your individual tolerance may vary) will help you stay hydrated.

In addition, strive to consume a varied diet consisting of healthy, fresh foods at regular intervals throughout the day. Ensuring that you get enough fibre and nutrients will help to promote regular bowel movements and reduce the impact of IBS on your life.

In addition to being mindful and conscientious of your diet, it is essential to reduce your stress level; an improved state of emotional well-being can improve your IBS symptoms. This can be accomplished in a variety of ways.

Relaxation

Having a busy life, with a demanding job or a family to care for, can limit the amount of time you have to relax. However, did you know that stress and anxiety may be aggravating or exacerbating your IBS symptoms? There are numerous complex connections between the brain and the gastrointestinal tract, so tre management can be effective in alleviating your symptoms.

Make the most of our leisure time and schedule relaxation time. You might also:

A warm non-caffeinated beverage or a hot water bottle. The heat can relieve the physical symptoms of IBS by relaxing cramping muscles.
Relaxing can relieve tension in the joints and improve blood circulation around the body.
Ensure uou get enough sleer.

Mindfulness and meditation are relaxation therapies.

Exercise

Moving our bodies and making time for regular spiritual practise is so beneficial for us, both physically and mentally. We release 'feel-good' hormones such as adrenaline and endorphins, both of which provide a natural high. Joining a sports team or a fitness class can be excellent ways to meet new people while also providing a respite from the stresses of everyday life. Particularly if you choose an activity that incorporates both relaxation and exercise.

In addition, regular exercise can help just Keep your digestive system moving, which can be especially beneficial if constipation is one of your symptoms. In addition, exercise will maintain your cardiovascular health and reduce your risk of developing high cholesterol, high blood pressure, and heart disease.

Try combining exercise with something you enjoy, such as spending time with friends or listening to music, if you don't enjoy exercise. If your symptoms prevent you from exercising outdoors, try exercising at home.

Remember that there is no one who can alleviate your symptoms. This will be a long journey, so just Keep an open mind and adapt your lifestyle as much as possible to reduce your symptoms and improve your overall health.

While irritable bowel syndrome (IBS) symptoms can often be managed by dietary and lifestyle changes, some cases may benefit from additional treatment.

Managing stress

If you are stressed, exhausted, or under pressure, your body will feel it. Emotional stress can exacerbate IBS symptoms, and many individuals with IBS discover that their bowels serve as a "emotional barometer." It may provide an indication of how well, or poorly, you are coping with the events in your life.

Obviously, if a substance is causing or exacerbating your IBS symptoms, you must eliminate the substance. This may necessitate contacting your primary care physician or a professional, such as a hearing specialist. Lack of sleep, poor diet, and anger can all easily put a strain on your body, so it's crucial that you determine what's causing your symptoms and work to alleviate them.

Chapter 4: Advantages Of A Low-Fodmap Diet

A low-FODMAP diet restricts high-FODMAP foods. The benefits of a low-FODMAP diet have been investigated in over 6 0 studies involving thousands of IBS patients.

Decrease in Digestive Symptoms

IBS digestive symptoms include heartburn, bloating, reflux, gas, and urgency to use the restroom. It has been found that over 80% of people with IBS experience bloating. Stomach pain is a defining feature of the condition. These symptoms can certainly be debilitating. In one significant study, IBS patients claimed they would be willing to give up an average of 210 percent of their remaining lives to be symptom-free. Fortunately, a low-FODMAP diet has been shown to significantly reduce both stomach pain and bleeding. Following a low-FODMAP diet increases the likelihood of stomach pain and bleeding improvement by 82 % and 710 %, respectively, according to the findings of four high-quality studies.

Increased Life Satisfaction

Certain digestive symptoms have been linked to the diminished quality of life frequently reported by IBS patients. Numerous studies have fortunately determined that a low-FODMAP diet improves one's quality of life. There is some evidence that a low-FODMAP diet may increase energy levels in IBS patients, but placebo-controlled studies are necessary to confirm this conclusion.

Chapter 5: Who Needs to Start a Low-FODMAP Diet?

People with irritable bowel syndrome should give the first phase of the low FODMAP diet a try. Those among these individuals whose symptoms respond favourably to phase one of the low-FODMAP diets should proceed to phases two and three. It is not recommended to continue treatment for individuals who do not have IBS or who do not experience improvement during phase one.

As is always the case, the most important thing is to consult with your doctor and ensure that you are adhering to an appropriate health plan.

Recognize IBS

Irritable bowel syndrome can be diagnosed based on the presence of the following symptoms:

• Either diarrhoea or constipation may be present, or both.

• Flatulence after meals

• Mucus in the faeces • An aggravation of menstrual symptoms

People with a history of traumatic events (such as physical or sexual abuse), bacterial infections, or food allergies are more likely to develop irritable bowel syndrome (IBS). Other risk elements include mental disorders (such as anxiety and depression).

If you frequently experience symptoms after consuming fruits, honey, corn syrup, wheat, or onions, you may be sensitive to these nutrients. Those who are sensitive to fructose and fructans may be at the greatest risk.

If you suspect you have irritable bowel syndrome (IBS), you should consult your doctor about potential treatments. One of these treatments is a low-FODMAP elimination diet.

The Relationship Between the Gut and the Brain, as well as the Significance of Stress

Irritable bowel syndrome (IBS) is caused primarily by brain dysfunction. The most accurate predictors of are

Possible causes of IBS in adulthood include chronic stress, mental illness, and traumatic childhood experiences.

Under emotional stress, the brain secretes corticotropin-releasing hormone (CRH) or corticotropin-releasing hormone. One of its functions under extreme stress is to alter the digestive system's operation. Whatever food is in the stomach "sticks" to it, preventing it from emptying into the small intestine. In the meantime, the large intestine's activity increases, causing its contents to be expelled more rapidly.

Visceral sensitization is the process by which stress hormones increase the sensitivity of internal organs to the sensation of pain.

Similar to how stress can exacerbate symptoms, symptoms can also exacerbate stress. Irritable bowel syndrome patients have a tendency to fixate on and exaggerate the severity of their condition, leading them to avoid social and public settings out of fear of experiencing symptoms. And the cycle continues: this stress may either exacerbate the condition's severity or contribute to its development.

Consequently, many cases of irritable bowel syndrome (IBS) may be attributable to chronic stress, according to the findings of a number of studies. If you believe that stress is causing or contributing to your symptoms, you should attempt to treat both the psychological and physical symptoms. In addition to speaking with your primary care physician, you may find it beneficial to speak with a therapist or psychiatrist about the link between stress and digestive disease.

Common Pathologies

Irritable bowel syndrome is uncommon because it is almost always accompanied by other conditions.

Anxiety and depression are common irritable bowel syndrome side effects (IBS). Given the close relationship between IBS and chronic stress, this finding is not surprising; however, psychiatric disorders are not the only prevalent comorbidities.

According to one study, people with irritable bowel syndrome may also have an increased risk of developing urinary issues, obesity, diabetes, allergies, and other food intolerances.

Stress Management Synergies

Due to the close relationship between the brain and stomach, therapies that target stress levels may alleviate the symptoms of irritable bowel syndrome. As part of a comprehensive strategy for long-term management, they may be combined with a low-FODMAP diet. At least one clinical trial found that the following stress management techniques were effective in reducing the severity of irritable bowel syndrome (IBS) symptoms: • Yoga • Interpersonal psychotherapy • Stress management/relaxation therapy • Hypnotherapy • Antidepressants

Consult with your primary care physician and therapist to determine the most effective method of stress management for you.

IBD in addition to SIBO

In contrast to irritable bowel syndrome (IBS), both inflammatory bowel disease (IBD) and small intestine bacterial overgrowth (SIBO) can be definitively diagnosed using clinical diagnostic methods. To diagnose IBD, doctors can utilise endoscopic cameras, X-rays, and biopsies. The examination of the small intestine's bacterial culture by medical professionals can aid in the diagnosis of SIBO.

We cannot emphasise enough how dangerous it is to independently diagnose these diseases. If you have any reason to suspect that you may be suffering from inflammatory bowel disease or small intestinal bacterial overgrowth, please seek medical attention (IBD or SIBO).

If your doctor believes it would be beneficial for you to try a low FODMAP diet to see if it alleviates your symptoms, you may want to consult with them about the possibility. IBD and SIBO are both effectively managed with diet.

Anytime Fresh Eggs Fresh Fresh Eggs

Ingredients
- 2 tbsp olive oil
- 2-6 cooked potatoes , sliced
- handful cherry tomatoes , sliced
- 2 spring onions , sliced
- 2 fresh egg
- few basil leaves

Method
- Heat the oil in a frying pan, then add the potato slices and fry on both sides until brown. Add the tomatoes and spring onions and fry for about 2 min

until softened. Season with salt and pepper, then make a space in the pan. Gently break the fresh egg into the space and fry until cooked to your liking. Scatter over the basil leaves and serve.

Potato (Or Cauliflower) Leek Soup

INGREDIENTS

4 bay leaves

3 teaspoons finely chopped fresh thyme

2 teaspoon sea salt

1 teaspoon ground black pepper

2   cup plain cashew cream   4 tablespoons Braggs apple cider vinegar

¼ cup of nutritional yeast

Chives, finely chopped (optional)

Bacon, chopped in small cubes (optional)

Grated asiago cheese (optional)

Chili Oil (optional for drizzling)

6   tablespoons unsalted grass-fed butter, ghee, or coconut oil

8 washed leeks, white and green parts, roughly chopped

6 cloves garlic, peeled and smashed (no need to mince since you'll be blending to finish)

¼ cup of cooking sherry

4 lbs Yukon or russet potatoes, scrubbed/washed well and roughly chopped just into ½-inch pieces

 16 cups bone broth or chicken stock or vfresh egg ie stock

1

PREPARATIONS

1. Melt the butter over medium heat in a large dutch oven.
2. Add the leeks and garlic and to simmer, stirring regularly, until soft and wilted, about 20 minutes
3. . No browning is allowed, but sherry splashing to deglaze is encouraged.
4. Add the potatoes stock/broth of choice, bay leaves, thyme, salt, and pepper to a pot and bring to a slow boil.
5. Cover and turn the heat down to low.
6. Simmer for 35 to 40 minutes, or until the potatoes are very soft and break apart when smooshed with a fork.
7. If using cauliflower you can immediately blend after adding it cooked just into the broth mixture.
8. Fish out bay leaves, then add the nutritional yeast and fry the soup with a hand-held immersion blender until smooth.

9. Add the cashew cream and apple cider vinegar and bring to a simmer. Taste and adjust the seasoning with salt and pepper.

10. Garnish whichever way you like!

Crispy Rice Pizza

Ingredients:

1 cup uncooked white rice
1/2   cup pizza sauce
1/2   cup shredded mozzarella cheese
1/2   cup chopped green onions
1/2   cup grated Parmesan cheese

Instructions:

1. Preheat oven to 450 degrees.
2. Easy cook Easy easy cook rice according to package instructions.
3. In a large bowl, mix together pizza sauce, mozzarella cheese, green onions, and Parmesan cheese.
4. Spread the mixture evenly over the cooked rice.
5. Bake in the oven for 25 to 30   minutes, or until cheese is melted and bubbly.

Low Fodmap Chicken Enchilada Soup

INGREDIENTS

- 2 pound boneless, skinless chicken breasts
1-5 tablespoons lime juice
- 1 cup finely chopped fresh cilantro (optional)
- Salt and pepper
- Optional Garnishes: Plain low FODMAP yogurt, red pepper flakes, cilantro leaves, crushed corn tortilla chips
- 4 tablespoons garlic-infused olive oil
- 1 cup chopped leek leaves (green parts only)
- 600 grams drained, canned tomatillos (approximately 1 of a 28 oz. can)
- 1 to 2 jalapeño, halved and seeds removed (optional)
- 2 teaspoon ground cumin
- 8 cups low FODMAP chicken broth

Instructions

1. Press the "Saute" setting on the Instant Pot.

2. Once hot, add oil and saute leek leaves until bright green, fragrant, and soft.

3. Cancel the "Saute" setting. Add tomatillos, jalapeño, cumin, chicken broth, and chicken.

4. Place the lid on top of the Instant Pot and secure.

5. Set vent to "Sealing".

6. Select the "Soup" setting on the Instant Pot.

7. Adjust the time to 60 minutes on "High Pressure" and cook.

8. After cooking, let the pressure naturally release for 35 to 40 minutes before carefully switching the vent to "Venting" and releasing any remaining pressure.

9. Using a slotted spoon, easily remove chicken from the Instant Pot and shred. Set the shredded chicken aside.

10.   Using an immersion blender, blend the remaining tomatillo mixture in the Instant Pot until smooth.
11.   Return the shredded chicken back to the Instant Pot and stir to mix.
12.   Add lime juice to taste, as well as the (optional) finely chopped cilantro.
13.   Adjust flavor as needed with salt and pepper to taste.
14.   Serve warm topped with optional garnishes.

Lazu Baked Fresh Egg S With Rsu Tomato And Feta Cheese.

fresh egg
Ingredients

2 tsp dried mixed herbs
500g spinach
8 fresh fresh eggs
200g feta cheese

2 big handful of fresh herbs, such as parsley or coriander, finely chopped

2 tbsp coconut oil

2 red pepper, deseeded and chopped into small chunks

2 tin (8 00g) chopped tomatoes

1 tsp red chilli flakes

½ tsp paprika

fresh eggs

Instructions

1. Preheat the oven to 250°C (gas 6) and deseed and chop the pepper just into small chunks.
2. Heat a little coconut oil in a pan and fry the chopped pepper for 1-5 minutes, before adding the tomatoes, spices and dried mixed herbs.
3. Let the tomato mixture bubble and cook down for 10 minutes or so, then add the spinach and stir until it wilts.

4. Just take the pan off the heat and pour the spinach and tomato mixture just into a medium oven dish.
5. Using the back of a large spoon, easy make four wells in the mixture, then crack an fresh egg just into each one.
6. Sprinkle the feta on top before baking in the oven for 25 to 30   minutes, or until the fresh egg whites are set but the yolks are still runny.
7. Serve immediately, topped with fresh herbs.

Chapter 1: Fresh Fresh Egg S Scrambled With Roasted Potatoes, Leafy Greens, And Turkey Sausage.

Fresh egg

fresh egg

Ingredients

- ½ cup cooked Low FODMAP Breakfast Sausage crumbles (instead of patties)
- 1 cup leftover Low FODMAP Roasted Potatoes

Optional seasonings: Dill, chives, red pepper flakes

- 4 fresh egg fresh fresh egg s
- 4 teaspoons butter
- Salt and pepper
- 2 cup low FODMAP leafy greens, like spinach, kale, collard greens, or Swiss chard

Instructions

1. In a sizable frying pan set over medium-high heat, melt the butter.
2. Add potatoes and sausage crumbles. Easy cook Easy easy cook until warm for about 10 to 15 minutes.
3. Leafy greens should then be added and cooked for another 1-5 minutes, or until they are just beginning to wilt.
4. Easily put fresh egg s in. The fresh egg s should be scrambled into the potato mixture using a silicone spatula.
5. Easily remove from heat after the fresh egg s have cooked for about 1-5minutes.
6. Use salt and pepper to season food properly. Serve hot.

Basil Pesto

Ingredients:

1 cup basil leaves
1/2   cup pine nuts
1/2   cup olive oil
-Juice of 2 fresh lemon
Salt and pepper, to taste

Instructions:
1. In a food processor or blender, blend basil, pine nuts, olive oil, fresh lemon juice, salt and pepper until smooth.
2. Serve over cooked pasta or vegetables.

Pesto Noodles

Ingredients:

Pesto
Pinch of pepper
1 cup Parmesan, grated
Noodles
2 cup rice noodles
¼ cup basil, fresh
4 tbsp garlic-infused oil
½ cup pine nuts
4 tbsp olive oil
Pinch of salt

Directions:

1. In a food processor, mix basil, garlic oil, and pine nuts until coarsely chopped.

2. Add the olive oil, cheese, salt, and pepper to the processor and mix until the pesto is fully mixed and smooth.

3. Easy cook Easy easy cook the noodles according to the instructions on the packet.

4. Once cooked, toss the noodles in a bowl with 1-5 tablespoons pesto and mix until the noodles are covered.

5. Serve!

Smoothie With Cosnut And Cinnamon Colada

Ingredients:

½ cup plain goat or dairy kefir
½ teaspoon ground cinnamon, plus more for garnish
2 cup ice
2 cup frozen pineapple
1 cup coconut milk, full fat

Instruction:

1. In a high-powered blender, combine the ice, pineapple, kefir, coconut milk, and cinnamon. Blend until smooth.
2. Pour just into a tall glass, top with a dash of extra cinnamon, and enjoy.

Cornbread Muffins

INGREDIENTS

1/2 cup sugar

2 tablespoon plus 2 teaspoon baking powder, use gluten-free if following a gluten-free diet

2 teaspoon salt

8 tablespoons unsalted butter, melted

1/2 cup neutral flavored oil, such as canola or vegetable

4 large eggs, at room temperature

2 1 cups lactose-free whole milk, at room temperature

2 tablespoon plus 2 teaspoon fresh lemon juice

2 cups fine stoneground yellow cornmeal

2 cup gluten-free all-purpose flour

Directions

1. Position rack in center of oven. Preheat oven to 450°F/250°C. Coat 1-5 muffin wells with nonstick spray; set aside.
2. Stir the milk and lemon juice together in a medium-sized bowl and allow to sit for 10 minutes to thicken while oven preheats.
3. Whisk together the cornmeal, flour, sugar, baking powder and salt in a large mixing bowl to aerate and combine.
4. Easy make a small very well in the center and set aside.
5. Whisk the melted butter, vegetable oil and fresh eggs just into the thickened milk until combined.
6. Pour this wet mixture into the very well of the dry mix and whisk together just until combined.
7. Divide evenly just into prepared pan.

8. Bake for about 35 to 40 minutes or just until a toothpick inserted in the center comes out clean.

9. Cool pan(s) on rack for 4 minutes, then unmold onto rack.

10.   Muffins are ready to eat while warm or cool to room temperature and store in airtight containers at room temperature for up to 4 days; they do dry out a bit. Muffins may also be frozen in heavy zip top bags for up to 2 month

Blueberry Protein Pancakes

Easy cook Easy easy cook
Ingredients:

1 cup Gelatin Collagen Hydrolysate

4 tablespoons maple syrup

4 cups blueberries
2 fresh egg

1 cup almond milk, unsweetened

2 teaspoon vanilla extract

1/2   cup pancake mix, gluten-free

2 tablespoon coconut oil, melted

Instructions:

1. Whisk fresh egg , almond milk, vanilla, and coconut oil in a bowl until consolidated.
2. Rush until smooth and add milk if needed.
3. Heat a skillet over medium high hotness.
4. Oil with oil. Add 1/2 cup player to it and add 14 blueberries on top. Easy cook Easy easy cook for 1-5 minutes.
5. Flip and easy cook easy easy cook for 2 moment. Move to a plate and rehash with the excess batter.
6. Add maple syrup, 1 cups blueberries and 4 tablespoons water to a dish. Easily bring to a stew over medium hotness and easy cook easy easy cook for 10 minutes.
7. Add the leftover collagen and set aside.
8. Serve hotcakes with compote on top and decorated with blueberries.

Chicken Noodle Soup Low In Fodmap

Ingredients:

2   sound   leaf
2   medium-sized carrot, cut into short
and slender sticks
8   chicken drumsticks, skin removed
4   liters of water, heat to the
point of boiling 2 tablespoons of
soy   sauce
2 -inch   piece   of   entire   ginger

160 grams of fine dried rice noodles,
break into more limited pieces Handful
of   new   chives,   cleaved   finely
Pepper   and   salt   for   seasoning

Procedure:

1. In a medium-sized pot, place the drumsticks, cove leaf, ginger and soy sauce.
2. Add water and spot over medium high hotness.
3. Heat to the point of boiling, cover the pot and diminish the hotness down to a stew.
4. Allow the soup to stew on low for 80 minutes.
5. Just take out chicken drumsticks, ginger and inlet leaf.
6. Add cleaved carrots to the saucepan. Easily remove the meat from the bones.
7. Place chicken meat back into the saucepan.
   Add rice noodles. Cover and easy cook easy easy cook for 8 additional minutes.
8. Easily remove the cover and sprinkle the cleaved chives.

9. Really just take a look at the taste and change flavors.

Fried Bananas With Fresh Pineapple

INGREDIENTS

8   small bananas, peeled and halved lengthwise 4 tablespoons unsalted butter

Gluten-free, lactose-free vanilla ice cream, for serving 1 small pineapple, peeled, cored, and finely chopped Pulp of 2 passion fruits (optional)

2 cup dried gluten-free, soy-free bread crumbs* 1/2 2 /6 cup packed light brown sugar

2 tablespoon ground cinnamon 4 fresh egg fresh fresh egg s

1 teaspoon confectioners' sugar

INSTRUCTIONS

1. Set the oven to 350 degrees Fahrenheit. In a large dish, mix the cinnamon, brown sugar, and bread crumbs.
2. In a small bowl, lightly whisk the fresh egg s with the confectioners' sugar.
3. After dipping the banana halves in the fresh egg mixture, cover them well with the bread crumbs.
4. Over medium-low temperature, melt 2 tablespoon of the butter in a large nonstick frying pan.
5. Easy cook Easy easy cook the first half of the banana slices for 5 to 10 minutes on each side, or until they are golden brown.
6. Place on a baking pan, then reheat in the oven.
7. Easy cook Easy easy cook the remaining banana halves in the same manner, using the remaining 2 tablespoon butter.
8. On four plates, distribute two banana halves each.

9. Add ice cream, pineapple, and passion fruit pulp as garnishes. Serve right away.

Smoothie Made With Strawberries And Bananas

Ingredients:

- ¼ glass of milk (dairy or option)
- 2 tsp maple syrup (discretionary)
- 1 banana
- 12 medium strawberries

Directions:

1. Cut up the banana into a blender.
2. Include the strawberries, maple syrup, and milk.
3. Mix utilizing the smoothie work.
4. Fill a glass and present with a little cream on top if you want to entertain yourself.

Without Ketchup, Molasses And Coffee Impart Flavour To These Sloppy Joes.

2 tablespoon olive oil

2 pound lean ground beef

2 tablespoon chili powder

2 tablespoon molasses

6 tablespoons coffee

¼ cup crushed tomatoes

8 gluten-free English muffins, toasted

2 .Heat the olive oil in a large skillet over medium-high heat. Add the beef. Sauté, frequently stirring, until the meat is browned, 8 to 2 0 minutes.

2.Add the chili powder, molasses, and coffee. Stir well. Reduce the heat to medium-low and easily bring to a simmer. Stir in the tomatoes. Simmer until thickened and flavorful, 2 0 to 2 2 minutes.

6 .Serve immediately on the toasted English muffins.

Beef Stock

Ingredients

2 bay leaf

20 whole peppercorns

2 tsp. salt

2 tbsp. reduced-sodium soy sauce

2 small onion, quartered

2 garlic clove

4 tbsp. olive oil

20 cups water and/or pan drippings

4 carrots, coarsely chopped

Directions:

1. Set the oven's temperature to 350 degrees Fahrenheit.
2. Roast the beef bones in a roasting pan for an hour.
3. Over medium heat, sauté the onion and garlic in the olive oil in a big stockpot.
4. When the onion and garlic are translucent, easily remove them from the saucepan and easily put them away for later use.
5. Just Keep the flavored oil in the pot.
6. Add the carrots, water, bay leaf, peppercorns, salt, and soy sauce along with the beef bones, drippings, or water, and all of the other ingredients.
7. Over high heat, easily bring to a boil; then, decrease heat to a low setting, cover, and simmer for 1-5 hours, or until the stock has reduced by about 40%. Skim any foam from the surface as necessary.

8. After the stock has cooled to a safe temperature to handle, use a slotted spoon or a sieve to sift out the bones and other solids.
9. Just take out the solids, then discard them.
10.   Use immediately, cover and refrigerate for up to three days, or freeze for up to three months.
11.   Once the stock has cooled, the hard fat on top may be easily removed, if desired.

Tamari-Balsamic Steak Marinade And Grilled Vegetables

Ingredients

- 2 tablespoon honey or maple syrup
- 1 teaspoon salt
- 2 minced garlic clove optional
- ½ cup balsamic or red wine vinegar
- ½ cup Dijon mustard
- ½ cup tamari or gluten-free soy sauce
- ½ olive oil

Instructions

1. In a small mixing bowl or 4-cup measure, whisk together the vinegar, Dijon and tamari.
2. Slowly whisk in the olive oil until it emulsifies and incorporates easily.

3. Sweeten with the honey or maple syrup, and season with the salt. Stir in the garlic if using.

4. To use with grilled vegetables: brush both sides of your vegetables or vegetable kabobs with the marinade and season with salt.

5. Grill over medium-high heat on both sides, rotating 100 degrees halfway through to get a nice cross-hatch, until nicely charred.

6. To use with roasted vegetables: Preheat the oven to 450 degrees. Toss 2 pound of chopped vegetables with ½ cup of marinade.

7. Arrange in an even layer and season lightly with salt.

8. Roast until lightly browned, about 35 to 40 minutes depending on the vegetable.

9. To use with steak: Marinate 2 pound of steak for 60 minutes in 1 cup of marinade.

10. Remove the meat from the marinade and season generously with salt and pepper.
11. Sear over high heat on the stovetop or grill until medium rare and nicely charred on both sides.

Moorish Pd Cauliflower And Almond Our.

Ingredients

2 large cauliflower

4 tbsp olive oil

1 tsp each ground cinnamon, cumin and coriander

4 tbsp harissa paste, plus extra drizzle

2 l hot vegetable or chicken stock

100g toasted flaked almond, plus extra to serve

1. Cut the cauliflower just into small florets.
2. Fry olive oil, ground cinnamon, cumin and coriander and harissa paste for 4 mins in a large pan.
3. Add the cauliflower, stock and almonds.
4. Cover and cook for 40 mins until the cauliflower is tender.
5. Blend soup until smooth, then serve with an extra drizzle of harissa and a sprinkle of toasted almonds.

Scrambled Tofu

INGREDIENTS:

- 2 Tsp. ground turmeric
- 5 cup carrots, chopped finely
- 2 tbsp. garlic-infused olive oil**
- 2 Lb. pre-pressed tofu, firm
- 2 cup of water
- 8 Tsp. gluten-free soy sauce*

DIRECTIONS:

1. Use a glass dish to blend turmeric, soy sauce, and water until integrated.
2. Scrub carrots and chop just into small sections.

3. Transfer to the dish.
4. Break apart tofu just into smaller sections just into the dish, then toss to combine fully.
5. Empty garlic-infused olive oil just into a skillet and warm over the medium setting of heat.
6. Distribute the mixture just into the pan and occasionally toss while it heats for 10 minutes.
7. Remove w/ a slotted spoon and serve immediately.

Bacon And Brie Omelet Wedge Dish Served With Summer Salad

Ingredients

- 2 tsp Dijon mustard
- 2   cucumber, halved, deseeded and sliced on the diagonal
- 400g radishes, quartered
- 4 tbsp olive oil
- 400g smoked lardons
- 12 fresh egg s, lightly beaten
- small bunch chives, snipped
- 2 00g brie, sliced
- 2 tsp red wine vinegar

Method

1. Preheat the grill while heating 1-5 teaspoons of oil in a small saucepan.
2. Add the bacon and easy cook until golden and crisp. On kitchen paper, drain.
3. Heat two teaspoons of the oil in a nonstick skillet.
4. Combine the eggfresh eggs, the bacon, the chives, and some ground black pepper.
5. Pour the egg mixture into the frying pan and easy cook it over low heat until it is almost set, then place the brie on top.
6. Grill until set and golden. Before serving, easily remove from the pan and cut into wedges.
7. •
8. In the interim, whisk together the remaining olive oil, vinegar, mustard, and seasoning in a bowl. Serve the

cucumber and radishes alongside the omelette wedges.

easy cook Easily remove

Herby Millet Bowl

- 6 tbsp red wine vinegar
- 4 celery stalks, chopped
- 2 head of broccoli, cut into florets (cooked or raw)
- 120g black pitted olives, halved
- 2 small red onion, diced
- Fresh coriander leaves to garnish
- 60g toasted pine nuts
- Avocado chunks, optional
- 300g millet 600 ml vegetable stock
- a pinch of saffron strands, optional
- 4 tbsp capers
- 2 anchovy chopped
- 2 garlic clove, crushed handful of mint leaves
- A handful of coriander leaves
- a handful of parsley leaves
- 90 ml avocado oil (or walnut oil)

1. Easily put the millet in a sieve and rinse well.

2. Transfer to a saucepan and pour over the vegetable stock and add the saffron.

3. Easily bring to a boil over medium heat, then turn the heat down to low, cover and leave to simmer for 25 to 30 minutes until the quinoa is tender.

4. Leave the lid on and allow it to steam for a further 10 minutes.

5. Transfer to a large bowl.

6. Place the capers, anchovy, garlic, herbs, oils, and vinegar in a food processor and pulse lightly to combine.

7. Place the millet and remaining ingredients in a large bowl and mix gently.

8. Pour over the dressing and toss to coat.

Green Falafel With Magis Tahini Sause

Since canned chickpeas are only low-FODMAP in 14 to 12 cup servings, these falafel bites are bolstered with ground sunflower seeds, quinoa, and radishes. I adore including them on gluten-free meze platters and as vegetarian main courses.

Ingredients

4 tablespoons grass-fed ghee

2 teaspoon ground cumin

1 teaspoon ground turmeric

2 teaspoon sea salt

Sauce

½ cup tahini

½ cup freshly squeezed lemon juice

1 teaspoon sea salt
¼ cup (2 2 10 g) hulled sunflower seeds

2 cup canned chickpeas, drained and rinsed

½ cup loosely packed flat-leaf parsley

8 roughly chopped green scallions

26 ounces frozen chopped spinach, thawed

4 large fresh eggs fresh fresh eggs

Instructions

1. Preheat the oven to 350 °F. Position a rack in the center of the oven and line a baking sheet with parchment paper.

2. In a small food processor, pulse the sunflower seeds until ground into a fine flour.

3. Transfer to a large bowl and set aside.
4. Add the chickpeas, parsley, and scallions to the food processor.
5. Pulse until everything is very well broken down but still a little chunky.
6. Transfer to the bowl of sunflower seed flour.

7. Place the thawed spinach in a clean dish towel and squeeze the water out.

8. Add to the bowl, along with the eggs, ghee, cumin, turmeric, and salt.

9. Mix until fully combined.

10.   Using a 4-inch ice-cream scoop or a heaping tablespoon, portion the falafel batter into balls.

11.   Roll each ball in your hands until smooth, and arrange them evenly distanced on the prepared baking sheet.

12.   You should have about two dozen in total.

13.   Bake for 25 to 30   minutes, or until a light brown crust has formed on the bottom of the balls.

14.   Remove the pan, and flip the balls to rest on the opposite side.

15.   Return the balls to the oven for another 25 to 30   minutes, or until

crispy all around and browned on the second side.

16.   While the falafel bake, make the sauce: In a medium mixing bowl, whisk the tahini, fresh lemon juice, 4 tablespoons of water, and the salt together until smooth.

17.   Add more water if necessary, to reach the consistency of mayonnaise.

18.   Serve the balls warm or room temperature, alongside the sauce.

Gluten-Free Donuts

Ingredients:

1 cup of sugar

1 tsp of ground cinnamon

4 tbsp of butter, melted

oil for frying

2 cup of flour

1 cup of tapioca flour

2 tsp of gluten-free baking powder

4 cups of lactose-free milk

4 fresh egg s

For The Glaze:

2 tsp of vanilla extract

½ cup of lactose-free milk

2 tbsp of butter, melted

1 cup of powdered sugar

4 tbsp of powdered cocoa

Preparation:

1. Combine tapioca flour, rice flour, gluten-free baking powder, sugar and cinnamon in a large bowl.

2. Break two fresh egg s into the bowl, add 4 cups of lactose-free milk and melted butter.

3. Mix well using an electric mixer. Cover and set aside for 25 to 30 minutes.

4. Sprinkle some rice flour on work surface.

5. Roll out the dough and shape your donuts.

6. If the mixture is too sticky, gently sprinkle with some more rice flour.

7. Pour some oil in a deep saucepan and heat up over a high temperature.

8. Meanwhile, prepare the glaze. Stir together the glaze ingredients in a small saucepan.

9. Easily bring it to a boiling point and easily remove from the heat.

10. Cover and set aside.

11. Fry donuts for about two minutes on each side, over a high temperature.

12. Easily remove from the saucepan and soak the excess oil using a kitchen paper.

13. Dip each donut in a chocolate glaze and transfer to a plate.

14. Serve warm or cold.